Those over 60 loose weight

You Can Achieve Your Weight Loss Goals After 60

By

Robert D. Fielder

Table of content

Introduction

As you get older, it can be more difficult to lose weight. This is because your metabolism slows down, and you may have more health conditions that make it harder to exercise. However, losing weight after 60 is still possible, and it can have several benefits for your health.

Losing weight after 60 can help you:

Reduce your risk of chronic diseases such as heart disease, stroke, type 2 diabetes, and some types of cancer.
Improve your blood pressure, cholesterol levels, and blood sugar levels.
Increase your energy levels.
Improve your sleep.
Improve your mood.
Increase your self-confidence.
If you are over 60 and you want to lose weight, there are several things you can do. Here are a few tips:

Eat a healthy diet. This means eating plenty of fruits, vegetables, and whole grains. It also means limiting your intake of processed foods, sugary drinks, and unhealthy fats.

Exercise regularly. Aim for at least 30 minutes of moderate-intensity exercise most days of the week.

Make lifestyle changes. This could include things like getting enough sleep, managing stress, and quitting smoking.

Losing weight after 60 can be challenging, but it is possible. By following these tips, you can improve your health and quality of life.

The Benefits of Losing Weight after 60

Losing weight after 60 can have several benefits for your health. These benefits include:

Reduced risk of chronic diseases: Losing weight can help reduce your risk of developing chronic diseases such as heart disease, stroke, type 2 diabetes, and some types of cancer.

Improved blood pressure, cholesterol levels, and blood sugar levels: Losing weight can help improve your blood pressure, cholesterol levels, and blood sugar levels. This can help reduce your risk of developing heart disease, stroke, and type 2 diabetes.

Increased energy levels: Losing weight can help increase your energy levels. This can make it easier to get through the day and enjoy your activities.

Improved sleep: Losing weight can help improve your sleep. This can help you feel more rested and alert during the day.

Improved mood: Losing weight can help improve your mood. This can help you feel happier and more positive about yourself.

Increased self-confidence: Losing weight can help increase your self-confidence. This can help you feel better about yourself and your appearance.

How to Set Realistic Goals

When you are setting goals for weight loss, it is important to set realistic goals. If you set unrealistic goals, you are more likely to give up. Here are a few tips for setting realistic goals:

Start by setting a small goal, such as losing 1-2 pounds per week.

Once you reach your first goal, you can set a new, slightly larger goal.

It is important to be patient and consistent with your weight loss efforts.
Remember that losing weight takes time and effort.
How to Stay Motivated

Losing weight can be challenging, but it is important to stay motivated. Here are a few tips for staying motivated:

Find a support system. Having people to support you can make a big difference.
Set realistic goals. As mentioned above, setting unrealistic goals can lead to discouragement and giving up.
Reward yourself for your progress. Rewarding yourself for your progress can help you stay motivated.
Don't give up. Losing weight takes time and effort, but it is possible.

Why weight loss after 60 is different

Metabolism: As you get older, your metabolism slows down. This means that you burn fewer calories at rest.

Muscle mass: As you get older, you lose muscle mass. Muscle tissue is metabolically active, so losing muscle mass can lead to a decrease in your metabolism.

Hormones: As you get older, your hormone levels can change. This can affect your appetite, energy levels, and metabolism.

Health conditions: As you get older, you may have more health conditions that can make it harder to lose weight. These conditions can include arthritis, heart disease, and diabetes.

Despite these challenges, it is still possible to lose weight after 60. Here are a few tips:

Eat a healthy diet. This means eating plenty of fruits, vegetables, and whole grains. It also means limiting your intake of processed foods, sugary drinks, and unhealthy fats.

Exercise regularly. Aim for at least 30 minutes of moderate-intensity exercise most days of the week.

Make lifestyle changes. This could include things like getting enough sleep, managing stress, and quitting smoking.

If you are over 60 and you want to lose weight, it is important to talk to your doctor. Your doctor can help you create a safe and effective weight loss plan.

Here are some additional tips for weight loss after 60:

Set realistic goals. Don't try to lose too much weight too quickly. Aim to lose 1-2 pounds per week.
Be patient. Losing weight takes time and effort. Don't get discouraged if you don't see results immediately.
Don't give up. Losing weight is a journey, not a destination. Keep at it and you will eventually reach your goals.
Sources:

The benefits of losing weight after 60

Reduced risk of chronic diseases: Losing weight can help reduce your risk of developing chronic diseases such as heart disease, stroke, type 2 diabetes, and some types of cancer.
Improved blood pressure, cholesterol levels, and blood sugar levels: Losing weight can help improve your blood pressure, cholesterol levels, and blood sugar levels. This can help reduce your risk of developing heart disease, stroke, and type 2 diabetes.

Increased energy levels: Losing weight can help increase your energy levels. This can make it easier to get through the day and enjoy your activities.

Improved sleep: Losing weight can help improve your sleep. This can help you feel more rested and alert during the day.

Improved mood: Losing weight can help improve your mood. This can help you feel happier and more positive about yourself.

Increased self-confidence: Losing weight can help increase your self-confidence. This can help you feel better about yourself and your appearance.

In addition to these health benefits, losing weight after 60 can also improve your quality of life. Losing weight can make it easier to do everyday activities, such as walking, bathing, and dressing. It can also make it easier to get around and enjoy your hobbies.

If you are over 60 and you want to lose weight, there are several things you can do. Here are a few tips:

Eat a healthy diet. This means eating plenty of fruits, vegetables, and whole grains. It also means limiting your intake of processed foods, sugary drinks, and unhealthy fats.

Exercise regularly. Aim for at least 30 minutes of moderate-intensity exercise most days of the week.
Make lifestyle changes. This could include things like getting enough sleep, managing stress, and quitting smoking.
If you are over 60 and you want to lose weight, it is important to talk to your doctor. Your doctor can help you create a safe and effective weight loss plan.

Here are some additional tips for weight loss after 60:

Set realistic goals. Don't try to lose too much weight too quickly. Aim to lose 1-2 pounds per week.
Be patient. Losing weight takes time and effort. Don't get discouraged if you don't see results immediately.
Don't give up. Losing weight is a journey, not a destination. Keep at it and you will eventually reach your goals.

How to set realistic goals

Start small. Don't try to lose too much weight too quickly. Aim to lose 1-2 pounds per week.

Be specific. Instead of saying "I want to lose weight," say "I want to lose 10 pounds in 3 months."

Make your goals measurable. How will you know if you have reached your goal? For example, you could say "I will lose 10 pounds if I weigh myself every week and track my progress."

Make your goals achievable. If you have never exercised before, don't set a goal of running a marathon. Start with something more achievable, like walking for 30 minutes a day.

Make your goals relevant. Your goals should be relevant to your lifestyle and your health goals. For example, if you have a family history of heart disease, you might set a goal of losing weight to reduce your risk of developing heart disease.

Make your goals time-bound. Give yourself a deadline for reaching your goal. This will help you stay motivated and on track.

By following these tips, you can set realistic goals that you are more likely to achieve.

Here are some additional tips for staying motivated:

Find a support system. Having people to support you can make a big difference. This could include friends, family, or a weight loss group.

Reward yourself for your progress. Rewarding yourself for your progress can help you stay motivated.
Don't give up. Losing weight takes time and effort, but it is possible. Keep at it and you will eventually reach your goals.

Chapter 1:

Diet

Eat plenty of fruits and vegetables. Fruits and vegetables are low in calories and high in nutrients. They are also a good source of fiber, which can help you feel full and satisfied.

Choose whole grains over processed grains. Whole grains are a good source of fiber and nutrients. Processed grains are often high in sugar and unhealthy fats.

Lean protein. Lean protein is a good source of protein and is low in fat. Good sources of lean protein include chicken, fish, beans, and lentils.

Healthy fats. Healthy fats are essential for good health. Good sources of healthy fats include olive oil, avocado, and nuts.

Limit unhealthy fats. Unhealthy fats are high in calories and can contribute to weight gain. Good sources of unhealthy fats include butter, margarine, and shortening.

Drink plenty of water. Water is essential for good health and can help you lose weight. Aim to drink eight glasses of water per day.

It is also important to be mindful of your portion sizes when you are trying to lose weight. Eating too much food can lead to weight gain, even if you are eating healthy foods. A good way to control your portion sizes is to use smaller plates and bowls. You can also eat slowly and savor your food. This will help you feel full before you overeat.

If you are struggling to eat a healthy diet, there are a few things you can do. First, talk to your doctor. Your doctor can help you create a healthy eating plan that is tailored to your individual needs. You can also talk to a registered dietitian. A registered dietitian is a trained professional who can help you make healthy food choices.

There are also several resources available online and in libraries that can help you learn more about healthy eating. The National Institutes of Health has a website called ChooseMyPlate.gov that provides information on healthy eating. The Mayo Clinic also has a website with information on healthy eating.

What to eat

Fruits and vegetables: Fruits and vegetables are low in calories and high in nutrients. They are also a good source of fiber, which can help you feel full and satisfied. Some good choices include apples, bananas, oranges, carrots, broccoli, and spinach.

Whole grains: Whole grains are a good source of fiber and nutrients. They are also a good source of complex carbohydrates, which can help you feel full and satisfied. Some good choices include brown rice, quinoa, and whole-wheat bread.

Lean protein: Lean protein is a good source of protein and is low in fat. Good sources of lean protein include chicken, fish, beans, and lentils.

Healthy fats: Healthy fats are essential for good health. Good sources of healthy fats include olive oil, avocado, and nuts.

Water: Water is essential for good health and can help you lose weight. Aim to drink eight glasses of water per day.

It is also important to be mindful of your portion sizes when you are trying to lose weight. Eating too much food can lead to weight gain, even if you are eating healthy foods. A good way to control your portion sizes is to use smaller plates and bowls. You can also eat slowly and savor your food. This will help you feel full before you overeat.

Here are some specific meal ideas that you can try:

Breakfast: Oatmeal with berries and nuts, yogurt with fruit, or eggs with whole-wheat toast.
Lunch: Salad with grilled chicken or fish, soup, or a sandwich on whole-wheat bread.
Dinner: Grilled chicken or fish with vegetables, brown rice, quinoa, or a tofu stir-fry.
If you are struggling to eat a healthy diet, there are a few things you can do. First, talk to your doctor. Your doctor can help you create a healthy eating plan that is tailored to your individual needs. You can also talk to a registered dietitian. A registered dietitian is a trained professional who can help you make healthy food choices.

There are also several resources available online and in libraries that can help you learn more about healthy eating. The National Institutes of Health has a website called ChooseMyPlate.gov that provides information on healthy eating. The Mayo Clinic also has a website with information on healthy eating.

What to avoid

Processed foods: Processed foods are often high in calories and low in nutrients. They also often contain unhealthy fats, sugar, and salt. Some examples of processed foods include chips, cookies, candy, and soda.

Sugary drinks: Sugary drinks are high in calories and low in nutrients. They can also contribute to weight gain and tooth decay. Some examples of sugary drinks include soda, juice, and sports drinks.

Fast food: Fast food is often high in calories and low in nutrients. It also often contains unhealthy fats, sugar, and salt. Some examples of fast food include burgers, fries, and pizza.

Alcohol: Alcohol is high in calories and can contribute to weight gain. It can also interfere with weight loss efforts.

Unhealthy fats: Unhealthy fats are high in calories and can contribute to weight gain. They can also increase your risk of heart disease and other health problems. Some examples of unhealthy fats include saturated fat and trans fat.

Salt: Salt can increase your risk of high blood pressure and other health problems. It is important to limit your intake of salt, especially if you have high blood pressure or other health problems.

It is also important to avoid eating too much food at any one time. Eating too much food can lead to weight gain, even if you are eating healthy foods. A good way to control your portion sizes is to use smaller plates and bowls. You can also eat slowly and savor your food. This will help you feel full before you overeat.

If you are struggling to avoid unhealthy foods, there are a few things you can do. First, talk to your doctor. Your doctor can help you create a plan to avoid unhealthy foods and reach your weight loss goals. You can also talk to a registered dietitian. A registered dietitian is a trained professional who can help you make healthy food choices.

There are also several resources available online and in libraries that can help you learn more about healthy eating. The National Institutes of Health has a website called ChooseMyPlate.gov that provides information on healthy eating. The Mayo Clinic also has a website with information on healthy eating.

How to create a healthy eating plan

Start by setting realistic goals. Don't try to change your entire diet overnight. Start by making small changes, such as adding more fruits and vegetables to your meals or cutting back on sugary drinks.

Make a list of healthy foods that you enjoy. This will make it easier to stick to your plan.

Plan your meals ahead of time. This will help you avoid unhealthy choices when you're hungry.

Cook more meals at home. This will give you more control over the ingredients in your food.

Read food labels carefully. This will help you make healthy choices when you're eating out.

Be patient. It takes time to change your eating habits. Don't get discouraged if you slip up. Just keep trying and you will eventually reach your goals.

Here are some specific meal ideas that you can try:

Breakfast: Oatmeal with berries and nuts, yogurt with fruit, or eggs with whole-wheat toast.

Lunch: Salad with grilled chicken or fish, soup, or a sandwich on whole-wheat bread.

Dinner: Grilled chicken or fish with vegetables, brown rice, quinoa, or a tofu stir-fry.

If you are struggling to create a healthy eating plan, there are a few things you can do. First, talk to your doctor. Your doctor can help you create a plan that is tailored to your individual needs. You can also talk to a registered dietitian. A registered dietitian is a trained professional who can help you make healthy food choices.

There are also several resources available online and in libraries that can help you learn more about healthy eating. The National Institutes of Health has a website called ChooseMyPlate.gov that provides information on healthy eating. The Mayo Clinic also has a website with information on healthy eating.

Chapter 2:

Exercise

There are many different types of exercise, so you can find something that you enjoy and that fits into your lifestyle. Some popular forms of exercise include:

Walking: Walking is a great way to get started with exercise. It's low-impact and easy on your joints. You can walk around your neighborhood, on a treadmill, or in a park.
Running: Running is a great way to burn calories and improve your cardiovascular health. If you're new to running, start slowly and gradually increase the distance and intensity of your runs.
Cycling: Cycling is a great way to get around town and enjoy the outdoors. It's also a low-impact exercise that's easy on your joints.
Swimming: Swimming is a great way to cool off on a hot day and get a full-body workout. It's also a low-impact exercise that's easy on your joints.

Yoga: Yoga is a great way to improve your flexibility, strength, and balance. It can also help reduce stress and improve your mood.

No matter what type of exercise you choose, it's important to start slowly and gradually increase the intensity and duration of your workouts. You should also talk to your doctor before starting any new exercise program, especially if you have any health conditions.

Here are some tips for getting started with exercise:

Set realistic goals. Don't try to do too much too soon. Start with a goal of exercising for 30 minutes three times a week.

Find an activity that you enjoy. If you don't enjoy your exercise, you're less likely to stick with it.

Make exercise a part of your routine. Schedule time for exercise in your day just like you would any other appointment.

Find a workout buddy. Having someone to exercise with can help you stay motivated.

Don't be afraid to ask for help. If you're not sure where to start, talk to a personal trainer or a certified fitness instructor.

The importance of exercise

Weight loss: Exercise can help you burn calories and lose weight.

Reduced risk of chronic diseases: Exercise can help reduce your risk of developing chronic diseases such as heart disease, stroke, type 2 diabetes, and some types of cancer.

Improved mood: Exercise can help improve your mood and reduce stress.

Increased energy levels: Exercise can help increase your energy levels and improve your sleep.

Stronger bones and muscles: Exercise can help strengthen your bones and muscles, which can help reduce your risk of injuries.

Improved balance and coordination: Exercise can help improve your balance and coordination, which can help reduce your risk of falls.

Improved mental health: Exercise can help improve your mental health by reducing stress, anxiety, and depression.

Increased lifespan: Exercise can help increase your lifespan.

If you are not used to exercising, start slowly and gradually increase the amount of exercise you do each week. It is also important to talk to your doctor before starting any new exercise program, especially if you have any health conditions.

There are many different types of exercise, so you can find something that you enjoy and that fits into your lifestyle. Some popular forms of exercise include:

Walking: Walking is a great way to get started with exercise. It's low-impact and easy on your joints. You can walk around your neighborhood, on a treadmill, or in a park.

Running: Running is a great way to burn calories and improve your cardiovascular health. If you're new to running, start slowly and gradually increase the distance and intensity of your runs.

Cycling: Cycling is a great way to get around town and enjoy the outdoors. It's also a low-impact exercise that's easy on your joints.

Swimming: Swimming is a great way to cool off on a hot day and get a full-body workout. It's also a low-impact exercise that's easy on your joints.

Yoga: Yoga is a great way to improve your flexibility, strength, and balance. It can also help reduce stress and improve your mood.

No matter what type of exercise you choose, it's important to start slowly and gradually increase the intensity and duration of your workouts. You should also talk to your doctor before starting any new exercise program, especially if you have any health conditions.

Here are some tips for getting started with exercise:

Set realistic goals. Don't try to do too much too soon. Start with a goal of exercising for 30 minutes three times a week.
Find an activity that you enjoy. If you don't enjoy your exercise, you're less likely to stick with it.
Make exercise a part of your routine. Schedule time for exercise in your day just like you would any other appointment.
Find a workout buddy. Having someone to exercise with can help you stay motivated.
Don't be afraid to ask for help. If you're not sure where to start, talk to a personal trainer or a certified fitness instructor.

What type of exercise is best for you?

Your fitness level: If you're new to exercise, start with something low-impact, like walking or swimming. As you get fitter, you can gradually increase the intensity and duration of your workouts.
Your interests: If you don't enjoy your exercise, you're less likely to stick with it. Find an activity that you find fun and challenging.
Your schedule: Make sure you can fit exercise into your schedule. If you have a busy lifestyle, choose an exercise that you can do at home or the gym during your lunch break.
Your budget: Some exercises, like yoga and Pilates, can be done at home without any equipment. Other exercises, like running and cycling, require you to purchase equipment.
Once you've considered these factors, you can start to narrow down your choices. Here are some popular types of exercise:

Walking: Walking is a great low-impact exercise that's easy on your joints. You can walk around your neighborhood, on a treadmill, or in a park.
Running: Running is a great way to burn calories and improve your cardiovascular health. If you're new to running, start slowly and gradually increase the distance and intensity of your runs.

Cycling: Cycling is a great way to get around town and enjoy the outdoors. It's also a low-impact exercise that's easy on your joints.

Swimming: Swimming is a great way to cool off on a hot day and get a full-body workout. It's also a low-impact exercise that's easy on your joints.

Yoga: Yoga is a great way to improve your flexibility, strength, and balance. It can also help reduce stress and improve your mood.

Pilates: Pilates is a great way to strengthen your core muscles. It can also help improve your flexibility and balance.

Weightlifting: Weightlifting is a great way to build muscle and strength. It can also help improve your bone health.

Martial arts: Martial arts is a great way to improve your fitness, coordination, and self-defense skills.

Dance: Dance is a great way to improve your fitness, coordination, and creativity.

No matter what type of exercise you choose, it's important to start slowly and gradually increase the intensity and duration of your workouts. You should also talk to your doctor before starting any new exercise program, especially if you have any health conditions.

Here are some tips for getting started with exercise:

Set realistic goals. Don't try to do too much too soon. Start with a goal of exercising for 30 minutes three times a week.
Find an activity that you enjoy. If you don't enjoy your exercise, you're less likely to stick with it.
Make exercise a part of your routine. Schedule time for exercise in your day just like you would any other appointment.
Find a workout buddy. Having someone to exercise with can help you stay motivated.
Don't be afraid to ask for help. If you're not sure where to start, talk to a personal trainer or a certified fitness instructor.

How much exercise do you need?

According to the Centers for Disease Control and Prevention (CDC), adults should aim for at least 150 minutes of moderate-intensity aerobic activity or 75 minutes of vigorous-intensity aerobic activity each week. This can be done in 30-minute increments on most days of the week. In addition, adults should do muscle-strengthening activities that work for all major muscle groups on two or more days a week.

Here are some examples of moderate-intensity aerobic activities:

Brisk walking
Biking
Swimming
Dancing
Water aerobics
Here are some examples of vigorous-intensity aerobic activities:

Running
Swimming laps
Jumping rope
Hiking
Playing basketball
If you are new to exercise, start slowly and gradually increase the amount of time you spend exercising. You should also talk to your doctor before starting any new exercise program, especially if you have any health conditions.

Here are some tips for getting started with exercise:

Set realistic goals. Don't try to do too much too soon. Start with a goal of exercising for 30 minutes three times a week.

Find an activity that you enjoy. If you don't enjoy your exercise, you're less likely to stick with it.

Make exercise a part of your routine. Schedule time for exercise in your day just like you would any other appointment.

Find a workout buddy. Having someone to exercise with can help you stay motivated.

Don't be afraid to ask for help. If you're not sure where to start, talk to a personal trainer or a certified fitness instructor.

an important part of a healthy lifestyle.

Chapter 3:

Lifestyle Changes

Lifestyle changes are changes that you make to your daily habits to improve your health. These changes can include things like eating a healthy diet, exercising regularly, getting enough sleep, and managing stress.

There are many benefits to making lifestyle changes. Eating a healthy diet can help you lose weight, reduce your risk of chronic diseases, and improve your mood. Exercising regularly can help you lose weight, improve your cardiovascular health, and reduce your risk of chronic diseases. Getting enough sleep can help you improve your mood, concentration, and memory. Managing stress can help you reduce your risk of chronic diseases and improve your overall health and well-being.

Making lifestyle changes can be challenging, but it is worth it for your health. There are many resources available to help you make lifestyle changes, such as your doctor, a registered dietitian, or a certified personal trainer.

Here are some tips for making lifestyle changes:

Start small. Don't try to change too much at once. Start with one or two changes and gradually add more as you become more comfortable.
Make sustainable changes. Choose changes that you can realistically stick with for the long term.
Find a support system. Having people to support you can make it easier to make lifestyle changes. Talk to your friends and family about your goals, and find a workout buddy or join a support group.
Don't give up. Making lifestyle changes takes time and effort. Don't get discouraged if you slip up. Just pick yourself up and keep going.
Making lifestyle changes can be a challenge, but it is worth it for your health. By following these tips, you can make lifestyle changes that will improve your health and well-being.

Here are some examples of lifestyle changes that can improve your health:

Eat a healthy diet. A healthy diet includes plenty of fruits, vegetables, and whole grains. It also limits processed foods, sugary drinks, and unhealthy fats.

Exercise regularly. Aim for at least 30 minutes of moderate-intensity exercise most days of the week.

Get enough sleep. Most adults need around 7-8 hours of sleep per night.

Manage stress. Find healthy ways to manage stress, such as exercise, yoga, or meditation.

Stress management

Stress is a normal part of life, but it can be harmful if it's not managed. There are many different ways to manage stress, and what works for one person may not work for another. Here are some tips for managing stress:

Identify your stressors. The first step to managing stress is to identify what's causing it. Once you know what your stressors are, you can start to develop strategies for dealing with them.

Take breaks. When you're feeling stressed, it's important to take breaks. Get up and move around, or step outside for some fresh air. Even a few minutes of relaxation can help to reduce stress levels.

Exercise. Exercise is a great way to relieve stress. It releases endorphins, which have mood-boosting effects. Aim for at least 30 minutes of moderate-intensity exercise most days of the week.

Get enough sleep. When you're sleep-deprived, you're more likely to feel stressed. Aim for 7-8 hours of sleep per night.

Eat a healthy diet. Eating a healthy diet can help to improve your mood and energy levels, which can make it easier to cope with stress. Avoid processed foods, sugary drinks, and unhealthy fats.

Practice relaxation techniques. Many different relaxation techniques can help to reduce stress, such as yoga, meditation, and deep breathing. Find a technique that works for you and practice it regularly.

Talk to someone. If you're feeling overwhelmed by stress, it can be helpful to talk to someone you trust, such as a friend, family member, therapist, or counselor. Talking about your problems can help you to feel better and develop coping strategies.

Sleep

Sleep is a state of rest in which the body and mind are inactive. During sleep, the body repairs itself and the brain processes information. Sleep is essential for good health and well-being.

There are many different stages of sleep, but they can be divided into two main categories: non-rapid eye movement (NREM) sleep and rapid eye movement (REM) sleep.

NREM sleep is divided into three stages: N1, N2, and N3. N1 is the lightest stage of sleep, and N3 is the deepest stage of sleep.
REM sleep is the stage of sleep in which most dreaming occurs.
Most adults need around 7-8 hours of sleep per night. However, some people may need more or less sleep. The amount of sleep you need depends on your age, lifestyle, and health.

If you don't get enough sleep, you may experience several problems, including:

Fatigue
Irritability
Difficulty concentrating

Increased risk of accidents
Increased risk of health problems, such as obesity, heart disease, and diabetes
There are many things you can do to improve your sleep. Here are a few tips:

Establish a regular sleep schedule and stick to it as much as possible, even on weekends. Go to bed and wake up at the same time each day, even on weekends. This will help to regulate your body's natural sleep-wake cycle.
Create a relaxing bedtime routine. This could include taking a warm bath, reading a book, or listening to calming music. Avoid watching TV or using electronic devices in the hour before bed, as the blue light emitted from these devices can interfere with sleep.
Make sure your bedroom is dark, quiet, and cool. Darkness helps to promote the production of melatonin, a hormone that helps to regulate sleep. Noise and light can disrupt sleep, so make sure your bedroom is as dark and quiet as possible. A cool temperature is also ideal for sleep.
Avoid caffeine and alcohol before bed. Caffeine and alcohol can interfere with sleep. Caffeine is a stimulant that can make it difficult to fall asleep.

Alcohol may help you fall asleep initially, but it can disrupt sleep later in the night.

Get regular exercise. Exercise can help to improve sleep quality. However, avoid exercising too close to bedtime, as this can make it difficult to fall asleep.

See a doctor if you have trouble sleeping. If you have trouble sleeping, talk to your doctor. There may be an underlying medical condition that is interfering with your sleep. Your doctor may be able to recommend treatment options to help you get a good night's sleep.

Managing medications

Managing medications can be a challenge, but it is important to take your medications as prescribed by your doctor to get the best results. Here are some tips for managing your medications:

Keep track of your medications. Make a list of all your medications, including the name, dosage, and frequency of each medication. You can keep this list in a notebook, on your phone, or in a medication organizer.

Take your medications on time. Set reminders on your phone or use a medication organizer to help you remember to take your medications on time.

Don't skip doses. Even if you're feeling better, it's important to take your medications as prescribed. Skipping doses can make your condition worse.

Don't double up on doses. If you forget to take a dose, don't double up on the next dose. Just take the next dose as scheduled.

Talk to your doctor if you have any questions or concerns about your medications. Your doctor can help you make sure you're taking your medications safely and effectively.

Here are some additional tips for managing medications:

Store your medications in a safe place. Keep your medications out of the reach of children and pets.

Do not take expired medications. Expired medications may not be effective or may even be harmful.

Dispose of your medications properly. Do not flush your medications down the toilet or pour them down the drain. Contact your local pharmacy or waste disposal company for instructions on how to properly dispose of your medications.

Chapter 4:

Staying Motivated

Staying motivated can be challenging, but there are a few things you can do to help yourself stay on track. Here are a few tips:

Set realistic goals. If your goals are too ambitious, you're more likely to get discouraged and give up. Start with small, achievable goals and gradually work your way up to bigger ones.

Break down your goals into smaller steps. This will make them seem less daunting and more manageable.

Reward yourself for your accomplishments. This will help you stay motivated and on track.

Find a support system. Having people to cheer you on and hold you accountable can make a big difference.

Don't be afraid to ask for help. If you're struggling, don't be afraid to ask for help from a friend, family member, therapist, or coach.

Here are some additional tips for staying motivated:

Visualize your success. Take some time to imagine yourself achieving your goals. This will help you stay focused and motivated.

Stay positive. It's important to stay positive and believe in yourself, even when things get tough.

Don't give up. Everyone has setbacks, but it's important to not give up on your goals. Keep working hard and you will eventually achieve them.

Staying motivated can be a challenge, but it's important to remember that you're not alone. Many people have been where you are and have successfully achieved your goals. By following these tips, you can help yourself stay on track and achieve your dreams.

How to stay on track

Staying on track can be a challenge, but there are a few things you can do to help yourself stay motivated and focused. Here are a few tips:

Set realistic goals. If your goals are too ambitious, you're more likely to get discouraged and give up. Start with small, achievable goals and gradually work your way up to bigger ones.

Break down your goals into smaller steps. This will make them seem less daunting and more manageable.

Reward yourself for your accomplishments. This will help you stay motivated and on track.

Find a support system. Having people to cheer you on and hold you accountable can make a big difference.

Don't be afraid to ask for help. If you're struggling, don't be afraid to ask for help from a friend, family member, therapist, or coach.

Here are some additional tips for staying on track:

Visualize your success. Take some time to imagine yourself achieving your goals. This will help you stay focused and motivated.

Stay positive. It's important to stay positive and believe in yourself, even when things get tough.

Don't give up. Everyone has setbacks, but it's important to not give up on your goals. Keep working hard and you will eventually achieve them.

Here are some specific strategies that can help you stay on track:

Make a plan. Once you know what you want to achieve, it's important to make a plan. This will help you stay focused and on track.

Set deadlines. Deadlines can help you stay motivated and on track.

Take action. Don't just sit around and wait for things to happen. Take action and make things happen.

Be flexible. Things don't always go according to plan. Be flexible and be willing to adjust your plans as needed.

Celebrate your successes. When you achieve a goal, take some time to celebrate your success. This will help you stay motivated and on track

Dealing with setbacks

Setbacks are a normal part of life. Everyone experiences them at some point. The important thing is to know how to deal with them healthily. Here are a few tips:

Allow yourself to feel your emotions. It's okay to feel disappointed, frustrated, or angry when you experience a setback. Don't try to bottle up your emotions. Allow yourself to feel them and then let them go.

Don't dwell on the past. It's important to learn from your setbacks, but don't dwell on them. Focus on the present and the future.

Don't give up on your goals. Just because you've experienced a setback doesn't mean you have to give up on your goals. Dust yourself off and keep going.

Ask for help. If you're struggling to deal with a setback, don't be afraid to ask for help from a friend, family member, therapist, or coach.

Here are some additional tips for dealing with setbacks:

Take some time for yourself. After a setback, it's important to take some time for yourself to relax and recharge. Do something you enjoy and that helps you to de-stress.

Talk to someone you trust. Talking to someone you trust about your setback can help you to process your emotions and feel supported.

Learn from your mistake. Every setback is an opportunity to learn and grow. Take some time to reflect on what went wrong and what you can do differently next time.

Don't be afraid to start over. If you've made a mistake, don't be afraid to start over. Everyone makes mistakes. The important thing is to learn from them and keep moving forward.

Celebrating your successes

Celebrating your successes is important because of it:

Boosts your confidence. When you take the time to celebrate your successes, you're sending a message to yourself that you're capable and worthy of success. This can help to boost your confidence and make you more likely to achieve your goals in the future.
Motivates you to keep going. When you see how far you've come, it can motivate you to keep going and achieve even greater things. Celebrating your successes can help you stay focused and motivated on your goals.
Makes you happier. Taking the time to celebrate your successes can simply make you feel good. It's a way to acknowledge your hard work and accomplishments, and it can help you feel more optimistic about your life.
There are many different ways to celebrate your successes. Here are a few ideas:

Treat yourself to something special. This could be anything from buying yourself a new outfit to going out to dinner.

Spend time with loved ones. Tell them how much you appreciate their support and celebrate your success with them.

Do something you enjoy. This could be anything from reading a book to going for a walk in nature.

Write down your accomplishments. This can help you to remember all of the great things you've achieved and keep you motivated to keep going.

Take a break. After all your hard work, take some time to relax and recharge. This could mean taking a nap, reading a book, or watching a movie.

Conclusion

The importance of lifelong weight management
Resources for further information
This table of contents provides a comprehensive overview of the topics that will be covered in the book. It is clear, concise, and easy to follow. It also includes information on the benefits of losing weight after 60, how to set realistic goals, and how to stay motivated. This book will be a valuable resource for anyone who is looking to lose weight after 60.

Here are some additional details that could be included in each chapter:

Chapter 1: Diet

Discuss the importance of eating a healthy diet that is rich in fruits, vegetables, and whole grains.
Provide tips on how to reduce your intake of processed foods, sugary drinks, and unhealthy fats.
Explain the importance of eating regular meals and snacks throughout the day.
Chapter 2: Exercise

Discuss the importance of regular exercise for weight loss and overall health.

Provide tips on how to choose the right type of exercise for you.

Explain how to gradually increase the intensity and duration of your workouts.

Chapter 3: Lifestyle Changes

Discuss the importance of managing stress, getting enough sleep, and managing medications.

Provide tips on how to make these changes in your life.

Chapter 4: Staying Motivated

Discuss the importance of setting realistic goals and celebrating your successes.

Provide tips on how to deal with setbacks.

This book will be a valuable resource for anyone who is looking to lose weight after 60. It provides comprehensive information on the topics of diet, exercise, lifestyle changes, and staying motivated.

Setbacks are a normal part of life. Everyone experiences them at some point. The important thing is to know how to deal with them healthily. Here are a few tips:

Allow yourself to feel your emotions. It's okay to feel disappointed, frustrated, or angry when you experience a setback. Don't try to bottle up your emotions. Allow yourself to feel them and then let them go.

Don't dwell on the past. It's important to learn from your setbacks, but don't dwell on them. Focus on the present and the future.

Don't give up on your goals. Just because you've experienced a setback doesn't mean you have to give up on your goals. Dust yourself off and keep going.

Ask for help. If you're struggling to deal with a setback, don't be afraid to ask for help from a friend, family member, therapist, or coach.

Here are some additional tips for dealing with setbacks:

Take some time for yourself. After a setback, it's important to take some time for yourself to relax and recharge. Do something you enjoy and that helps you to de-stress.

Talk to someone you trust. Talking to someone you trust about your setback can help you to process your emotions and feel supported.

Learn from your mistake. Every setback is an opportunity to learn and grow. Take some time to reflect on what went wrong and what you can do differently next time.

Don't be afraid to start over. If you've made a mistake, don't be afraid to start over. Everyone makes mistakes. The important thing is to learn from them and keep moving forward.

Setbacks can be tough, but they don't have to stop you from achieving your goals. By following these tips, you can learn to deal with setbacks healthily and come out stronger on the other side.

Celebrating your successes is also important because of it:

Boosts your confidence. When you take the time to celebrate your successes, you're sending a message to yourself that you're capable and worthy of success. This can help to boost your confidence and make you more likely to achieve your goals in the future.

Motivates you to keep going. When you see how far you've come, it can motivate you to keep going and achieve even greater things. Celebrating your successes can help you stay focused and motivated on your goals.

Makes you happier. Taking the time to celebrate your successes can simply make you feel good. It's a way to acknowledge your hard work and accomplishments, and it can help you feel more optimistic about your life.

There are many different ways to celebrate your successes. Here are a few ideas:

Treat yourself to something special. This could be anything from buying yourself a new outfit to going out to dinner.

Spend time with loved ones. Tell them how much you appreciate their support and celebrate your success with them.

Do something you enjoy. This could be anything from reading a book to going for a walk in nature.

Write down your accomplishments. This can help you to remember all of the great things you've achieved and keep you motivated to keep going.

Take a break. After all your hard work, take some time to relax and recharge. This could mean taking a nap, reading a book, or watching a movie.

No matter how you choose to celebrate your successes, make sure to take the time to do it. It's important to acknowledge your hard work and accomplishments, and celebrating your successes is a great way to do that.

Thanks for reading my book